The Comprehensive Ketogenic Diet Delicacies

An Essential Step-By-Step Cooking Guide to Burn Fat and Boost Your Energy

Michelle Lewis

Contents

Vanilla Butter Cake

Preparation Time: 10 minutes

Cooking Time: 35 minutes

Servings: 9

Ingredients:

- 5 eggs
- 1 tsp. baking powder
- Oz. almond flour
- 1/2 cup butter, softened
- 1 cup Swerve
- 4 oz. cream cheese, softened
- 1 tsp. vanilla
- 1 tsp. orange extract

Directions:

1. Turn the oven on and preheat to 350 F/ 180C. Spray 9-inch cake pan with cooking spray and set aside. Add all ingredients into the mixing bowl and whisk until batter is fluffy. Bake for 35-40 minutes. Slices and serve.

Nutrition:

289 Calories

27.2g Total Fat

2.2g Fiber

Carrot Cake

Preparation Time: 10 minutes

Cooking Time: 35 minutes

Servings: 16

Ingredients:

- 2 eggs
- ½ tsp. vanilla
- 2 tbsp. butter, melted
- ½ cup carrots, grated
- 1/8 tsp. ground cloves
- 1 tsp. cinnamon
- 1 tsp. baking powder
- 2 tbsp. unsweetened shredded coconut
- ¼ cup pecans, chopped
- 6 tbsp. erythritol
- ¾ cup almond flour
- Pinch of salt

Directions:

1. Start oven and preheat to 325 F/ 162 C. Spray cake pan with cooking spray and set aside. Whisk cloves, cinnamon, baking powder, almond flour, shredded coconut, nuts, sweetener, and salt.

2. Stir in eggs, vanilla, butter, and shredded coconut until well combined. Bake for 30-35 minutes. Slice and serve.

Nutrition:

111 Calories

10.6g Total Fat

1.6g Fiber

Delicious Almond Cake

Preparation Time: 10 minutes

Cooking Time: 40 minutes

Servings: 16

Ingredients:

- 4 eggs
- 1 tsp. baking powder
- 1 1/2 tsp. vanilla
- 1/3 cup Swerve
- 2 oz. cream cheese, softened
- 2 tbsp. butter
- 1 cup almond flour
- 1/2 cup coconut flour
- 4 oz. half and half
- Pinch of salt

For topping:

- 3/4 cup almonds, toasted and sliced
- 1/3 cup Swerve
- 6 tbsp. butter, melted
- 1 cup almond flour

Directions:

1. Turn the oven on and preheat to 350 F/ 180C. Spray 8-inch cake pan with cooking spray and set aside. Add all ingredients except topping

ingredients into the large bowl whisk until well combined.

2. Pour batter into the prepared cake pan and spread evenly. Combine all topping ingredients. Sprinkle topping mixture evenly on top of batter.

3. Bake for 40 minutes. Remove from oven and allow cooling completely. Slice and serve.

Nutrition:

198 Calories

18.2g Total Fat

5.9g Protein

Lemon Cheesecake

Preparation Time: 10 minutes

Cooking Time: 55 minutes

Servings: 8

Ingredients:

- 4 eggs
- 18 oz. ricotta cheese
- 1 fresh lemon zest
- 2 tbsp. swerve
- 1 fresh lemon juice

Directions:

1. Turn the oven on and preheat to 350 F/ 180C. Spray cake pan with cooking spray and set aside. Beat ricotta cheese until smooth.
2. Add egg one by one and whisk well. Add lemon juice, lemon zest, and swerve and mix well. Transfer mixture into the prepared cake pan and bake for 50-55 minutes.
3. Remove cake from oven and set aside to cool completely. Place cake in the fridge for 1-2 hours. Slice and serve.

Nutrition:

12 Calories

7.3g Total Fat

10.2g Protein

Delicious Cheesecake

Preparation Time: 15 minutes

Cooking Time: 70 minutes

Servings: 8

Ingredients:

- 3 eggs
- 1/4 cup shredded coconut
- 1/2 cup coconut flour
- 1/2 cup almond flour
- 1 tsp. vanilla
- 1 tbsp. stevia
- 15.5 oz. sour cream
- 8 oz. cream cheese, softened
- 1/2 cup butter, melted

Directions:

1. Start to preheat oven 150 C. Grease 9-inch spring-form pan with cooking spray. Set aside.
2. For the crust
3. In a mixing bowl, mix together coconut flour, almond flour, shredded coconut, and melted butter until well combined. Transfer crust mixture into the prepared pan and spread evenly and press down with a fingertip. Place pan into the fridge to set crust.

4. For the cheesecake filling

5. In a large bowl, beat sour cream and cream cheese together. Add egg, vanilla, and sweetener and beat until well combined. Pour cheesecake filling evenly over crust. Place pan in a water bath and bake for 1 hour-1 hour 20 minutes. Remove cake pan from oven and set aside to cool completely.

6. Place cake pan into the fridge for 5-6 hours. Slice and serve.

Nutrition:

410 Calories

39g Total Fat

7.8g Protein

Pumpkin Cheesecake

Preparation Time: 15 minutes

Cooking Time: 80 minutes

Servings: 8

Ingredients:

For Crust:

- 1/2 cup almond flour
- 1 tbsp. swerve
- 1/4 cup butter, melted
- 1 tbsp. flaxseed meal

For Filling:

- 3 eggs
- 1/2 tsp. ground cinnamon
- 1/2 tsp. vanilla
- 2/3 cup pumpkin puree
- 15.5 oz. cream cheese
- 1/4 tsp. ground nutmeg
- 2/3 cup Swerve
- Pinch of salt

Directions:

1. Start to preheat oven to 300 F. Coat 9-inch spring-form pan with cooking spray. Set aside.
2. For Crust:

3. In a bowl, mix together almond flour, swerve, flaxseed meal, and salt. Add melted butter and mix well to combine. Transfer crust mixture into the prepared pan and press down evenly with a fingertip. Bake for 10-15 minutes. Allow to cool for 10 minutes.

4. For the cheesecake filling:

5. In a large bowl, beat cream cheese until smooth and creamy. Add eggs, vanilla, swerve, pumpkin puree, nutmeg, cinnamon, and salt and stir until well combined.

6. Pour cheesecake batter into the prepared crust and spread evenly. Bake for 50-55 minutes. Remove cheesecake from oven and set aside to cool completely. Place cheesecake in the fridge for 4 hours. Slices and serve.

Nutrition:

320 Calories

30.4g Total Fat

8.2g Protein

Flourless Chocó Cake

Preparation Time: 10 minutes

Cooking Time: 45 minutes

Servings: 8

Ingredients:

- 7 oz. unsweetened dark chocolate, chopped
- ¼ cup Swerve
- 4 eggs, separated
- 6 oz. cream
- 6 oz. butter, cubed

Directions:

1. Grease 8-inch cake pan with butter and set aside. Add butter and chocolate in microwave safe bowl and microwave until melted. Stir well. Add sweetener and cream and mix well.
2. Add egg yolks mix until combined. Beat egg whites in another bowl. Fold egg whites to the chocolate mixture. Bake at 325 F/ 162 C for 45 minutes. Slice and serve.

Nutrition:

318 Calories

28.2g Total Fat

6.6g Protein

Gooey Chocolate Cake

Preparation Time: 10 minutes

Cooking Time: 20 minutes

Servings: 8

Ingredients:

- 2 eggs
- 1/4 cup unsweetened cocoa powder
- 1/2 cup almond flour
- 1/2 cup butter, melted
- 1 tsp. vanilla
- 3/4 cup Swerve
- Pinch of salt

Directions:

1. Turn the oven on and preheat to 350 F/ 180C. Spray 8-inch spring-form cake pan with cooking spray. Set aside. In a bowl, sift together almond flour, cocoa powder, and salt. Mix well and set aside.

2. In another bowl, whisk eggs, vanilla extract, and sweetener until creamy. Slowly fold the almond flour mixture into the egg mixture and stir well to combine. Add melted butter and stir well.

3. Pour cake batter into the prepared pan and
   bake for 20 minutes. Remove from oven and
   allow cooling completely. Slice and serve.

Nutrition:

166 Calories

16.5g Total Fat

3.5g Protein

Coconut Cake

Preparation Time: 10 minutes

Cooking Time: 20 minutes

Servings: 8

Ingredients:

- 5 eggs, separated
- ½ tsp. baking powder
- ½ tsp. vanilla
- ½ cup butter softened
- ½ cup erythritol
- ¼ cup unsweetened coconut milk
- ½ cup coconut flour
- Pinch of salt

Directions:

1. Start to preheat oven to 400 F/ 200 C. Grease cake pan with butter and set aside. In a bowl, beat sweetener and butter until combined. Add egg yolks, coconut milk, and vanilla and mix well.

2. Add baking powder, coconut flour, and salt and stir well. In another bowl, beat egg whites until stiff peak forms. Gently fold egg whites into the cake mixture.

3. Pour batter in a prepared cake pan and bake in preheated oven for 20 minutes. Slice and serve.

Nutrition:

163 Calories

16.2g Total Fat

3.9g Protein

Peach Cake

Preparation Time: 10 minutes

Cooking Time: 20 minutes

Servings: 12

Ingredients:

- 6 eggs
- 2 peaches, stoned, cut into quarters
- 1 tsp. vanilla extract
- 1 tsp. baking powder
- 9 ounces almond meal
- 4 Tbsp. Swerve
- A pinch of salt
- 2 Tbsp. orange zest
- 2 ounces stevia
- 4 ounces cream cheese
- 4 ounces plain Greek yogurt

Directions:

1. Pulse peaches in a food processor. Add Swerve, almond meal, eggs, baking powder, vanilla extract, a pinch of salt, and pulse well. Transfer into 2 spring form pans.
2. Place in an oven at 350F and bake for 20 minutes. In a bowl, mix cream cheese with yogurt, orange zest, stevia, and stir well. Place

one cake layer on a plate. Then add half of the cream cheese mixture, add the other cake layer

3. Then top with the rest of the cream cheese mixture. Spread it well. Slice and serve.

Nutrition:

207 Calories

16.5g Fat

8.7g Protein

Chocolate Chip Cookie

Preparation Time: 15 minutes

Cooking Time: 1 minute

Servings: 14

Ingredients

Balls

- 1 cup almond flour
- ½ teaspoon vanilla extract
- 1 tablespoon powdered swerve sweetener
- ¼ cup dark chocolate chips
- ¼ cup heavy cream

Chocolate Ganache

- 1 ½ tablespoon dark chocolate
- 1 tablespoon unsalted butter

Directions

1. Mix flour in it, add vanilla, sweetener, and cream.
2. Fold in chocolate chips, and shape the mixture into balls.
3. Melt chocolate and butter in microwave for 1 minute, stir every 15 seconds.
4. Drizzle chocolate over the balls, rest for 5 minutes and serve.

Nutrition

74 Calories

7g Fat

2g Protein

Cream Cheese Fudge

Preparation Time: 4 hours

Cooking Time: 2 minutes

Servings: 24

Ingredients

- 2 ounces chocolate
- ½ cup powdered stevia
- 1 tablespoon vanilla extract
- ½ cup salted butter
- 8 ounces cream cheese, full-fat

Directions

1. Melt chocolate and butter for 2 minutes stir every 30 seconds.
2. Whisk sweetener and vanilla using an electric blender
3. Mix cream cheese in it, pour in chocolate mixture, using hand whisk.
4. Take a 6-by-8-inch pan, grease it with oil, spoon the chocolate mixture, and spread evenly.
5. Freeze 4 hours, then cut and serve.

Nutrition

145 Calories

13.6g Fat

2.9g Protein

Blueberry Ice Pops

Preparation Time: 5 minutes

Cooking Time: 20 minutes

Servings: 4

Ingredients

- 3 ounces fresh blueberries
- 35 drops of liquid stevia
- 1 tablespoon lemon juice
- 1 cup coconut milk

Directions

1. Blend all the ingredients in food processor.
2. Pour the mixture into ice pop molds and freeze for 6 hours.
3. Dip each pop mold into hot water to release.

Nutrition

154 Calories

15.2g Fat

3.2g Protein

Blueberry Crisp

Preparation Time: 5 minutes

Cooking Time: 20 minutes

Servings: 2

Ingredients

- 1/8 cup almond flour
- 1 cup fresh blueberries
- 2 tablespoons powdered swerve sweetener
- ¼ cup pecan halves
- 1 tablespoon ground flax
- ¼ teaspoon salt
- ½ teaspoon ground cinnamon
- ½ teaspoon vanilla extract
- 2 tablespoons unsalted butter
- 2 tablespoons heavy cream

Directions

1. Preheat oven to 400°F.
2. Fill each ramekin with ½ cup berries and ½ tablespoon sweetener, and stir.
3. Blend remaining ingredients into a food processor, spoon this mixture over berries.
4. Bake for 20 minutes, top each with 1 tablespoon of heavy cream.

Nutrition

390 Calories

35g Fat

6g Protein

Chocolate Chaffles

Preparation Time: 10 minutes

Cooking Time: 20 minutes

Servings: 4

Ingredients

- ½ cup chocolate chips
- ¼ cup swerve sweetener
- 1 teaspoon vanilla extract
- ½ cup unsalted butter
- 3 eggs, room temperature

Directions

1. Preheat according to the manufacturer's instructions.
2. Melt butter and chocolate chips, for 1 minute.
3. Whisk eggs, mix vanilla and sweetener then whisk in chocolate.
4. Grease the waffle maker with avocado oil spray and pour prepared batter.
5. Close waffle maker and cook for 8 minutes.
6. When done, remove by using a tong repeat with the remaining batter.

Nutrition

672 Calories

70g Fat

13g Protein

Almond Cookies

Preparation Time: 10 minutes

Cooking Time: 20 minutes

Servings: 18

Ingredients

2 tbsp. Almond butter

1 tbsp. Coconut oil

¼ cup Coconut milk

2 tbsp. Sugar-free coconut syrup

2 large Eggs

½ tsp. Baking powder

½ tsp. Salt

2 tbsp. Granulated sugar substitute

1 ½ cup Sugar-free dried coconut

½ cup Flax meal

2 squares 90% dark chocolate

18 Almonds

Directions:

In a bowl, combine the coconut oil and almond butter and mix well.

Add the eggs, syrup, and coconut milk and mix until smooth.

Stir in the flax meal, dried coconut, sweetener, salt, and baking powder.

Roll the dough into 18 (1-inch) balls and place on a parchment covered cookie sheet.

Press lightly to make a dent on each ball.

Top with chopped chocolate (each cookie) and top with an almond.

Bake in a preheated 375F/190C oven until browned and slightly puffed, about 20 minutes.

Serve.

Nutrition:

Calories 114

Fat 11g

Carb 4g

Protein 3g

Pumpkin Pie Cupcakes

Preparation Time: 15 minutes

Cooking Time: 30 minutes

Servings: 6

Ingredients

3 Tbsp. Coconut flour

1 tsp. Pumpkin pie spice

¼ tsp. Baking powder

¼ tsp. Baking soda

Pinch salt

¾ cup Pumpkin puree

1/3 cup Swerve brown

¼ cup Heavy whipping cream

1 Egg

½ tsp. Vanilla

Directions:

Line 6 muffin cups with parchment paper and preheat the oven to 350F.

In a bowl, whisk together the salt, baking soda, baking powder, pumpkin pie spice, and coconut flour.

In another bowl, whisk egg, vanilla, cream, sweetener, and pumpkin puree until mixed. Whisk in dry ingredients.

Pour into the muffin cups and bake until just puffed and almost set, about 25 to 30 minutes.

Remove and cool.

Refrigerate for about 1 hour.

Top with whipped cream and serve.

Nutrition:

Calories: 70

Fat: 4.1g

Carb: 5.1g

Protein: 1.7g

Brownies

Preparation Time: 15 minutes

Cooking Time: 20 minutes

Servings: 16

Ingredients

½ cup, melted Butter.

2/3 cup Swerve sweetener

3 Eggs

½ tsp. Vanilla extract

½ cup Almond flour

1/3 cup Cocoa powder

1 Tbsp. Gelatin

½ tsp. Baking powder

¼ tsp. Salt

¼ cup Water

1/3 cup Sugar-free chocolate chips

Directions:

Grease a (8 x 8-inch) baking pan and preheat the oven to 350F.

In a bowl, whisk together eggs, vanilla extract, sweetener, and butter.

Add the salt, baking powder, gelatin, cocoa powder, and flour and whisk until combined. Stir in the chocolate chips.

Fill the prepared baking pan with the batter.

Bake until center still a bit wet, but the edges are set, about 15 to 20 minutes.

Remove, cool, slice, and serve.

Nutrition:

Calories: 110

Fat: 9.5g

Carb: 3.6g

Protein: 3.1g

Ice Cream

Preparation Time: 15 minutes

Cooking Time: 30 minutes

Servings: 8

Ingredients

2 ½ cups, divided Heavy whipping cream.

¼ cup Swerve brown

¼ cup Sugar substitute

2 Tbsp. Butter

1 ½ tsp. Maple extract

¼ tsp. Xanthan gum

1/3 cup Chopped walnuts.

Directions:

In a saucepan, bring two sweeteners, and 1 ¼ cups of the whipping cream to a simmer. Lower heat and gently simmer for 30 minutes.

Remove from the heat and whisk in maple extract, and butter. Add the xanthan gum and whisk to mix well. Cool, and then place in the refrigerator for about 2 hours.

Beat the remaining whipping cream in a bowl until stiff peaks. Foil in chilled cream/maple until well combined. Stir in chopped walnuts.

Freeze until firm.

Serve.

Nutrition:

Calories: 318

Fat: 31.7g

Carb: 2.9g

Grilled cheese chaffle

Preparation time: 3 minutes

Cooking time: 8 *minutes*

Servings: 1

Ingredients:

1 egg

1/4 teaspoon garlic powder

1/2 cup shred cheddar

2 american cheese or 1/4 cup shredded cheese

1 tablespoon butter

Directions

 In a small bowl, mix bacon, garlic powder and shredded cheddar cheese.

After heating the dash waffle maker, add half the mixture of the scramble. Cook and cook for 4 minutes.

Add to the dash mini waffle maker the remainder of the scramble mixture and cook for 4 minutes.

Steam the stove pan over moderate heat when both chaffles are finished.

Attach 1 spoonful of butter and dissolve. Place one chaffle in the pan once the butter has melted. Place your favorite cheese on top of the chaffle and finish with a second chaffle.

Cook the chaffle for 1 minute on the first side, turn it over and cook for another 1-2 minutes on the other side to finish the cheese melting.

Cut it from the bread when the cheese melts and eat it!

Nutrition:

Calories: 549kcal

carbohydrates: 3g

protein: 27g

fats: 48g

 saturated fats: 28g

cholesterol: 295mg

sodium: 1216mg

potassium: 172mg

sugar: 1g

Baked potato chaffle using jicama

Servings: 1

Ingredients: 1 jicama root

1/2 onion, medium, minced

2 cloves garlic, pressed - 1 cup cheese

1 eggs, whisked - Salt and pepper

Directions:

Peel the jicama root and shred it using a food processor.

Place the shredded jicama root in a colander to allow the water to drain. Mix in 2 tsp of salt as well.

Squeeze out the remaining liquid.

Microwave the shredded jicama for 5-8 minutes. This step pre-cooks it.

Mix all the remaining Ingredients together with the jicama. Start preheating the waffle maker. Once preheated, sprinkle a bit of cheese on the waffle maker, allowing it to toast for a few seconds. Place 3 tbsp of the jicama mixture onto the waffle maker. Sprinkle more cheese on top before closing the lid. Cook for 5 minutes. Flip the chaffle and let it cook for 2 more minutes.

Servings your baked jicama by topping it with sour cream, cheese, bacon pieces, and chives.

Nutrition: calories: 168 carbohydrates: 5.1g fat: 11.8g protein: 10g

Fried pickle chaffle sticks

Servings: 1

Ingredients:

1 egg

1/2 cup mozzarella cheese

1/4 cup pork panko

6-8 pickle slices, thinly sliced

1 tbsp pickle juice

Directions:

Mix all the Ingredients, except the pickle slices, in a small bowl.

Use a paper towel to blot out excess liquid from the pickle slices.

Add a thin layer of the mixture to a preheated waffle iron.

Add some pickle slices before adding another thin layer of the mixture.

Close the waffle maker's lid and allow the mixture to cook for 4 minutes.

Optional: combine hot sauce with ranch to create a great-tasting dip.

Nutrition:

calories: 465

carbohydrate: 3.3g

fat: 22.7g

protein: 59.2g

Tiramisu chaffle

Servings: 8

Ingredients:

2 eggs

2 oz cream cheese, softened

1 tbsp coconut flour

1 tbsp heavy cream

1 tsp vanilla extract

1/2 tsp baking powder

1/2 tsp ground cinnamon

1/4 tsp stevia powder

For the coffee syrup:

4 tbsp strong coffee

5 drops liquid stevia

For the filling:

1 oz cream cheese, softened

3 oz mascarpone cheese, softened

1/4 cup heavy cream

2 tsp vanilla extract

1/4 tsp stevia powder

For dusting:

1/2 tsp unsweetened cocoa powder

Directions:

Preheat the mini waffle maker.

Combine all the chaffle Ingredients in a blender.

Once the waffle maker is heated, pour about 1/4 of the batter and allow it to cook for 5-6 minutes. Remove the cooked chaffle and repeat this step for the remaining batter.

While waiting for the chaffle to cook, mix the liquid stevia and coffee in a small bowl for the coffee syrup.

For the filling, mix the vanilla, stevia powder, and heavy cream. Whisk this until soft peaks start to form.

In a separate mixing bowl, use a hand mixer to combine the mascarpone and cream cheese. Once done, mix it in with the whipped cream.

To assemble, drizzle 1 tbsp of coffee syrup on the chaffle.

On one chaffle, spread a quarter of the filling. Top this with another chaffle, and repeat the previous step until you have four layers of chaffles.

Dust the finished tiramisu chaffle with the unsweetened cocoa powder.

Refrigerate this for 6 hours or more before serving.

Nutrition: calories: 567 carbohydrate: 6.6g

fat: 53.4g protein: 14.7g

Spicy jalapeno popper chaffles

Servings: 1

Ingredients: for the chaffles:

1 egg

1 oz cream cheese, softened

1 cup cheddar cheese, shredded

For the toppings:

2 tbsp bacon bits

1/2 tbsp jalapenos

Directions:

Turn on the waffle maker. Preheat for up to 5 minutes.

Mix the chaffle Ingredients.

Pour the batter onto the waffle maker.

Cook the batter for 3-4 minutes until it's brown and crispy.

Remove the chaffle and repeat steps until all remaining batter have been used up.

Sprinkle bacon bits and a few jalapeno slices as toppings.

Nutrition:

calories: 231

carbohydrate: 2g

fat: 18g

protein: 13g

Breakfast chaffle sandwich

Servings: 1

Ingredients:

1 egg

1/2 cup monterey jack chee cse

1 tbsp almond flour

2 tbsp butter

Directions:

Preheat the waffle maker for 5 minutes until it's hot.

Combine monterey jack cheese, almond flour, and the egg in a bowl. Mix well.

Take 1/2 of the batter and pour it into the preheated waffle maker. Allow to cook for 3-4 minutes.

Repeat previous step for the remaining batter.

Melt butter on a small pan. Just like you would with french toast, add the chaffles and let each side cook for 2 minutes. To make them crispier, press down on the chaffles while they cook.

Remove the chaffles from the pan. Allow to cool for a few minutes. Servings.

Nutrition: calories: 514 carbohydrates: 2g fat: 47g protein: 21g

Peanut butter and

jelly chaffles

Servings: 1

Ingredients: 1 egg

2 slices cheese, thinly sliced

1 tsp natural peanut butter

1 tsp sugar-free raspberr y preServings

Cooking spray

Directions:

Crack and whisk the egg in a small bowl or a measuring cup.

Lightly grease the waffle maker with Cooking spray.

Preheat the waffle maker.

Once it is heated up, place a slice of cheese on the waffle maker and wait for it to melt.

Once melted, pour the egg mixture onto the melted cheese.

Once the egg starts cooking, carefully place another slice of cheese on the waffle maker.

Close the lid. Cook for 3-4 minutes.

Take out the chaffles and place on a plate.

Top the chaffles with whipped cream.

Drizzle some natural peanut butter and raspberry preServings on top.

Nutrition: calories: 337 carbohydrates: 3g fat: 27g protein: 21g

Halloumi cheese chaffles

Servings: 1

Ingredients:

3 oz halloumi cheese

2 tbsp pasta sauce

Directions:

Make half-inch thick slices of halloumi cheese.

With the waffle maker still turned off, place the cheese slices on it.

Turn on the waffle maker and let the cheese cook for 3-6 minutes.

Remove from the waffle maker and let it cool.

Add low-carb pasta or marinara sauce.

Nutrition:

calories: 333

carbohydrates: 2g

fat: 26g

protein: 22g

Chaffles benedict

Servings: 4

Ingredients: for the chaffles:

12 eggs

1 cup cheddar cheese, shredded

8 slices bacon

For the hollandaise sauce:

3 egg yolks

1 tbsp lemon juice

2 pinches kosher salt

1/4 tsp dijon mustard or hot sauce, optional

1/2 cup butter, salted

Directions:

Preheat the waffle maker.

Pour water in a pan and place over medium-high heat.

Take 4 eggs and beat them in a bowl. The remaining eggs are for poaching.

Once the waffle maker is heated up, sprinkle 1 tbsp of cheese and allow it to toast.

Take 1 1/2 tbsp of the beaten eggs and place on the toasted cheese.

Once the egg starts cooking, add another layer of sprinkled cheese on top.

Close the lid. Cook for 2-3 minutes.

Remove the cooked chaffle and repeat the steps until you've created 8 chaffles.

Fry bacon and set aside for later.

Poach the remaining eggs.

To make the sauce, combine lemon juice, salt, egg yolks, and dijon mustard or hot sauce in a bowl.

In a separate container, melt the butter in the microwave. Let it cool for a few minutes.

Pour the melted butter over the egg yolk mixture.

Using an immersion blender, pulse the mixture until it becomes yellow and cloudy. Continue pulsing until the consistency becomes creamy and thick.

To Servings, place cooked chaffles on a plate.

Place a slice of bacon over each chaffle.

Top the bacon with poached egg and drizzle with hollandaise sauce.

Nutrition:

calories: 601

carbohydrates: 1g

fat: 51g

protein: 34g

Carnivore chaffle

Servings: 1

Ingredients: 1 egg

1/3 cup mozzarella cheese

1/2 cup pork rinds - Salt

Directions: Preheat the waffle maker.

In a small mixing bowl, mix a pinch of salt with the cheese, egg, and pork rinds.

Pour the mixture onto the preheated waffle maker. Close the lid and wait for 3-5 minutes while it cooks. You'll know it's cooked once it already has a golden-brown color.

Carefully remove it from the waffle maker and Servings.

Nutrition: calories: 274 carbohydrates: 1g

fat: 20g protein: 23g

Eggnog chaffles

Servings: 1

Ingredients: 1 egg, separated

1 egg yolk - 1 tsp coconut flour

1/2 cup mozzarella che ese, shredded

1/2 tsp spiced rum - 1 tsp vanilla extract

1/4 tsp nutmeg, dried

A dash of cinnamon

For the icing:

2 tbsp cream cheese

1 tbsp powdered sweetener

2 tsp rum or rum extract

Directions:

Preheat the mini waffle maker.

Mix egg yolk in a small bowl until smooth.

Add in the sweetener and mix until the powder is completely dissolved.

Add the coconut flour, cinnamon, and nutmeg. Mix well.

In another bowl, mix rum, egg white, and vanilla. Whisk until well combined.

Throw in the yolk mixture with the egg white mixture. You should be able to form a thin batter.

Add the mozzarella cheese and combine with the mixture. Separate the batter into two batches. Put 1/2 of the batter into the waffle maker and let it cook for 6 minutes until it's solid.

Repeat until you've used up the remaining batter.

In a separate bowl, mix all the icing Ingredients.

Top the cooked chaffles with the icing, or you can use this as a dip.

Nutrition: calories: 266 carbohydrates: 2g

fat: 23g protein: 13g

Cheddar jalapeno chaffles

Servings: 1

Ingredients:

1 egg

1/2 cup cheddar chee se, shredded

1 tbsp almond flour

1 tbsp jalapenos

1 tbsp olive oil

Directions:

Preheat the waffle maker.

While waiting for the waffle maker to heat up, mix jalapeno, egg, cheese, and almond flour in a small mixing bowl.

Lightly grease the waffle maker with olive oil.

In the center of the waffle maker, carefully pour the chaffle batter. Spread the mixture evenly toward the edges.

Close the waffle maker lid and wait for 3-4 minutes for the mixture to cook. For an even crispier texture, wait for another 1-2 minutes.

Remove the chaffle. Let it cool before serving.

Nutrition:

calories: 509

carbohydrates: 5g

fat: 45g

protein: 23g

Cauliflower chaffle

Preparation time: 5 minutes

Cooking time: 5 *minutes*

Servings: 1

Ingredients:

1/2 cup of rice cauliflower

1/4 shredded cheddar

1 large egg from which half of the yolk has been removed

1 tbsp fine almond flour

Salt and pepper

Sprinkle extra cheese on the bottom.

Directions

 spread the mix on a waffle iron and add more cheese.

Cook for 8 minutes.

Note: when immersed in ketchup, it tastes like a hash brown. Oh, it cuts the cheese in half nutrition value

Calories 200

16g fat

11g protein

4g total carbs

2g pure carbohydrate

Fiber2g

Sugar 0g

Buffalo hummus beef chaffles

Preparation time: 15 minutes

Cooking time: 32 minutes

Servings: 4

Ingredients:

2 eggs

1 cup + ¼ cup finely grated cheddar cheese, divided

2 chopped fresh scallions

Salt and freshly ground black pepper to taste

2 chicken breasts, cooked and diced

¼ cup buffalo sauce

3 tbsp low-carb hummus

2 celery stalks, chopped

¼ cup crumbled blue cheese for topping

Directions:

Preheat the waffle iron.

In a medium bowl, mix the eggs, 1 cup of the cheddar cheese, scallions, salt, and black pepper,

Open the iron and add a quarter of the mixture. Close and cook until crispy, 7 minutes.

Transfer the chaffle to a plate and make 3 more chaffles in the same manner.

Preheat the oven to 400 f and line a baking sheet with parchment paper. Set aside.

Cut the chaffles into quarters and arrange on the baking sheet.

In a medium bowl, mix the chicken with the buffalo sauce, hummus, and celery.

Spoon the chicken mixture onto each quarter of chaffles and top with the remaining cheddar cheese.

Place the baking sheet in the oven and bake until the cheese melts, 4 minutes.

Remove from the oven and top with the blue cheese.

Servings afterward.

Nutrition: Calories 552 Fats 28.37g

carbs 6.97g net carbs 6.07g protein 59.8g

Pulled pork chaffle sandwiches

Preparation time: 20 minutes

Cooking time: 28 minutes

Servings: 4

Ingredients:

2 eggs, beaten

1 cup finely grated cheddar cheese

¼ tsp baking powder

2 cups cooked and shredded pork

1 tbsp sugar-free bbq sauce

2 cups shredded coleslaw mix

2 tbsp apple cider vinegar

½ tsp salt

¼ cup ranch dressing

Directions:

Preheat the waffle iron.

In a medium bowl, mix the eggs, cheddar cheese, and baking powder.

Open the iron and add a quarter of the mixture. Close and cook until crispy, 7 minutes.

Transfer the chaffle to a plate and make 3 more chaffles in the same manner.

Meanwhile, in another medium bowl, mix the pulled pork with the bbq sauce until well combined. Set aside.

Also, mix the coleslaw mix, apple cider vinegar, salt, and ranch dressing in another medium bowl.

When the chaffles are ready, on two pieces, divide the pork and then top with the ranch coleslaw. Cover with the remaining chaffles and insert mini skewers to secure the sandwiches.

Enjoy afterward.

Nutrition:

Calories 374

Fats 23.61g carbs 8.2g net carbs 8.2g protein 28.05g

Okonomiyaki chaffles

Preparation time: 20 minutes

Cooking time: 28 minutes

Servings: 4

Ingredients:

For the chaffles: 2 eggs, beaten

1 cup finely grated mozzarella cheese

½ tsp baking powder

¼ cup shredded radishes

For the sauce: 2 tsp coconut aminos

2 tbsp sugar-free ketchup

1 tbsp sugar-free maple syrup

2 tsp worcestershire sauce

For the topping: 1 tbsp mayonnaise

2 tbsp chopped fresh scallions

2 tbsp bonito flakes

1 tsp dried seaweed powder

1 tbsp pickled ginger

Directions:

For the chaffles:

Preheat the waffle iron. In a medium bowl, mix the eggs, mozzarella cheese, baking powder, and radishes. Open the iron and add a quarter of the mixture. Close and cook until crispy, 7 minutes.

Transfer the chaffle to a plate and make a 3 more chaffles in the same manner.

For the sauce: Combine the coconut aminos, ketchup, maple syrup, and worcestershire sauce in a medium bowl and mix well.

For the topping:

In another mixing bowl, mix the mayonnaise, scallions, bonito flakes, seaweed powder, and ginger

To Servings:

Arrange the chaffles on four different plates and swirl the sauce on top. Spread the topping on the chaffles and Servings afterward.

Nutrition: Calories 90 Fats 3.32g carbs 2.97g net carbs 2.17g protein 12.09g

Ketogenic reuben chaffles

Preparation time: 15 minutes

Cooking time: 28 minutes

Servings: 4

Ingredients:

For the chaffles: 2 eggs, beaten

1 cup finely grated swiss cheese

2 tsp caraway seeds - 1/8 tsp salt

½ tsp baking powder

For the sauce: 2 tbsp sugar-free ketchup

3 tbsp mayonnaise - 1 tbsp dill relish

1 tsp hot sauce

For the filling:

6 oz pastrami

2 swiss cheese slices

¼ cup pickled radishes

Directions:

For the chaffles:

Preheat the waffle iron.

In a medium bowl, mix the eggs, swiss cheese, caraway seeds, salt, and baking powder.

Open the iron and add a quarter of the mixture. Close and cook until crispy, 7 minutes.

Transfer the chaffle to a plate and make 3 more chaffles in the same manner.

For the sauce:

In another bowl, mix the ketchup, mayonnaise, dill relish, and hot sauce.

To assemble:

Divide on two chaffles; the sauce, the pastrami, swiss cheese slices, and pickled radishes.

Cover with the other chaffles, divide the sandwich in halves and Servings.

Nutrition:

Calories 316 Fats 21.78g carbs 6.52g net carbs 5.42g protein 23.56g

Pumpkin-cinnamon churro sticks

Preparation time: 10 minutes

Cooking time: 14 minutes

Servings: 2

Ingredients: 3 tbsp coconut flour

¼ cup pumpkin puree - 1 egg, beaten

½ cup finely grated mozzarella cheese

2 tbsp sugar-free maple syrup + more for serving

1 tsp baking powder

1 tsp vanilla extract

½ tsp pumpkin spice seasoning

1/8 tsp salt

1 tbsp cinnamon powder

Directions:

Preheat the waffle iron. Mix all the Ingredients in a medium bowl until well combined. Open the iron and add half of the mixture. Close and cook until golden brown and crispy, 7 minutes.

Remove the chaffle onto a plate and make 1 more with the remaining batter.

Cut each chaffle into sticks, drizzle the top with more maple syrup and Servings after.

Nutrition: Calories 219 Fats 9.72g carbs 8.64g net carbs 4.34g protein 25.27g

Low carb Ketogenic broccoli cheese waffles

Preparation time: 5 minutes

Cooking time: 5 *minutes*

Servings: 2

Ingredients:

1 cup broccoli, processed

1 cup shredded cheddar cheese

1/3 cup grated parmesan cheese

2 eggs, beats

Directions

spray the Cooking spray on the waffle iron and preheat.

Use a powerful blender or food processor to process the broccoli until rice consistency.

Mix all Ingredients in a medium bowl.

Add 1/3 of the mixture to the waffle iron and cook for 4-5 minutes until golden.

Nutritional value

Calories 160 Total fat 11.8g 18%

Cholesterol 121mg 40% Sodium 221.8mg 9%

Total carbohydrate 5.1g 2%

Dietary fiber 1.7g 7%

Sugars 1.2g Protein 10g 20%

Vitamin a 133.5µg 9%

Vitamin c 7.3mg 12%

Guacamole chaffle bites

Preparation time: 10 minutes

Cooking time: 14 minutes

Servings: 2

Ingredients:

1 large turnip, cooked and mashed

2 bacon slices, cooked and finely chopped

½ cup finely grated monterey jack cheese

1 egg, beaten

1 cup guacamole for topping

Directions:

Preheat the waffle iron.

Mix all the Ingredients except for the guacamole in a medium bowl.

Open the iron and add half of the mixture. Close and cook for 4 minutes. Open the lid, flip the chaffle and cook further until golden brown and crispy, 3 minutes.

Remove the chaffle onto a plate and make another in the same manner.

Cut each chaffle into wedges, top with the guacamole and Servings afterward.

Nutrition:

Calories 311

Fats 22.52g carbs 8.29g net carbs 5.79g protein 13.62g

Zucchini parmesan chaffles

Preparation time: 10 minutes

Cooking time: 14 minutes

Servings: 2

Ingredients:

1 cup shredded zucchini

1 egg, beaten

½ cup finely grated parmesan cheese

Salt and freshly ground black pepper to taste

Directions:

Preheat the waffle iron.

Put all the Ingredients in a medium bowl and mix well.

Open the iron and add half of the mixture. Close and cook until crispy, 7 minutes.

Remove the chaffle onto a plate and make another with the remaining mixture.

Cut each chaffle into wedges and Servings afterward.

Nutrition:

Calories 138

Fats 9.07g carbs 3.81g net carbs 3.71g protein 10.02g

Blue cheese chaffle bites

Preparation time: 10 minutes

Cooking time: 14 minutes

Servings: 2

Ingredients:

1 egg, beaten

½ cup finely grated parmesan cheese

¼ cup crumbled blue cheese

1 tsp erythritol

Directions:

Preheat the waffle iron.

Mix all the Ingredients in a bowl.

Open the iron and add half of the mixture. Close and cook until crispy, 7 minutes.

Remove the chaffle onto a plate and make another with the remaining mixture.

Cut each chaffle into wedges and Servings afterward.

Nutrition:

Calories 196

Fats 13.91g carbs 4.03g net carbs 4.03g protein 13.48g

Chaffle fruit snacks

Preparation time: 10 minutes

Cooking time: 14 minutes

Servings: 2

Ingredients:

1 egg, beaten

½ cup finely grated cheddar cheese

½ cup greek yogurt for topping

8 raspberries and blackberries for topping

Directions:

Preheat the waffle iron.

Mix the egg and cheddar cheese in a medium bowl.

Open the iron and add half of the mixture. Close and cook until crispy, 7 minutes.

Remove the chaffle onto a plate and make another with the remaining mixture.

Cut each chaffle into wedges and arrange on a plate.

Top each waffle with a tablespoon of yogurt and then two berries.

Servings afterward.

Nutrition:

Calories 207

Fats 15.29g carbs 4.36g net carbs 3.86g protein 12.91g

Ketogenic belgian sugar chaffles

Preparation time: 10 minutes

Cooking time: 24 minutes

Servings: 4

Ingredients:

1 egg, beaten

2 tbsp swerve brown sugar

½ tbsp butter, melted

1 tsp vanilla extract

1 cup finely grated parmesan cheese

Directions:

Preheat the waffle iron.

Mix all the Ingredients in a medium bowl.

Open the iron and pour in a quarter of the mixture. Close and cook until crispy, 6 minutes.

Remove the chaffle onto a plate and make 3 more with the remaining Ingredients.

Cut each chaffle into wedges, plate, allow cooling and Servings.

Nutrition:

Calories 136

Fats 9.45g carbs 3.69g net carbs 3.69g protein 8.5g

Lemon and paprika chaffles

Preparation   time: 10   minutes

 Cooking   time: 28   minutes

  Servings: 4

Ingredients:

1 egg, beaten

1 oz cream cheese, softened

1/3 cup finely grated m ozzarella cheese

1 tbsp almond flour

1 tsp butter, melted

1 tsp maple (sugar-free) syrup

½ tsp sweet paprika

½ tsp lemon extract

Directions:

Preheat the waffle iron.

Mix all the Ingredients in a medium bowl

Open the iron and pour in a quarter of the mixture. Close and cook until crispy, 7 minutes.

Remove the chaffle onto a plate and make 3 more with the remaining mixture.

Cut each chaffle into wedges, plate, allow cooling and Servings.

Nutrition: Calories 48 Fats 4.22g carbs 0.6g net carbs 0.5g protein 2g

Herby chaffle snacks

Preparation time: 10 minutes

Cooking time: 28 minutes

Servings: 4

Ingredients:

1 egg, beaten

½ cup finely grated monter ey jack cheese

¼ cup finely grated parmesan cheese

½ tsp dried mixed herbs

Directions:

Preheat the waffle iron.

Mix all the Ingredients in a medium bowl

Open the iron and pour in a quarter of the mixture. Close and cook until crispy, 7 minutes.

Remove the chaffle onto a plate and make 3 more with the rest of the Ingredients.

Cut each chaffle into wedges and plate.

Allow cooling and Servings.

Nutrition:

Calories 96

Fats 6.29g carbs 2.19g net carbs 2.19g protein 7.42g

Pumpkin spice chaffles

Preparation time: 10 minutes

Cooking time: 14 minutes

Servings: 2

Ingredients:

1 egg, beaten

½ tsp pumpkin pie spice

½ cup finely grated mozzarella cheese

1 tbsp sugar-free pumpkin puree

Directions:

Preheat the waffle iron.

In a medium bowl, mix all the Ingredients.

Open the iron, pour in half of the batter, close, and cook until crispy, 6 to 7 minutes.

Remove the chaffle onto a plate and set aside.

Make another chaffle with the remaining batter.

Allow cooling and Servings afterward.

Nutrition:

Calories 90

Fats 6.46g carbs 1.98g net carbs 1.58g protein 5.94g

Breakfast spinach
ricotta chaffles

Preparation time: 10 minutes

Cooking time: 28 minutes

Servings: 4

Ingredients:

4 oz frozen spinach, thawed, squeezed dry

1 cup ricotta cheese

2 eggs, beaten

½ tsp garlic powder

¼ cup finely grated pecorino romano cheese

½ cup finely grated mozzarella cheese

Salt and freshly ground black pepper to taste

Directions:

Preheat the waffle iron.

In a medium bowl, mix all the Ingredients.

Open the iron, lightly grease with Cooking spray and spoon in a quarter of the mixture.

Close the iron and cook until brown and crispy, 7 minutes.

Remove the chaffle onto a plate and set aside.

Make three more chaffles with the remaining mixture.

Allow cooling and Servings afterward.

Nutrition: Calories 188 Fats 13.15g carbs 5.06g net carbs 4.06g protein 12.79g

Scrambled egg

stuffed chaffles

Preparation time: 15 minutes

Cooking time: 28 minutes

Servings: 4

Ingredients:

For the chaffles:

1 cup finely grated chedda r cheese

2 eggs, beaten

For the egg stuffing:

1 tbsp olive oil

4 large eggs

1 small green bell pepper, deseeded and chopped

1 small red bell pepper, deseeded and chopped

Salt and freshly ground black pepper to taste

2 tbsp grated parmesan cheese

Directions:

For the chaffles:

Preheat the waffle iron.

In a medium bowl, mix the cheddar cheese and egg.

Open the iron, pour in a quarter of the mixture, close, and cook until crispy, 6 to 7 minutes.

Plate and make three more chaffles using the remaining mixture.

For the egg stuffing:

Meanwhile, heat the olive oil in a medium skillet over medium heat on a stovetop.

In a medium bowl, beat the eggs with the bell peppers, salt, black pepper, and parmesan cheese.

Pour the mixture into the skillet and scramble until set to your likeness, 2 minutes.

Between two chaffles, spoon half of the scrambled eggs and repeat with the second set of chaffles.

Servings afterward.

Nutrition:

Calories 387

Fats 22.52g carbs 18.12g net carbs 17.52g protein 27.76g

Mixed berry-vanilla chaffles

Preparation time: 10 minutes

Cooking time: 28 minutes

Servings: 4

Ingredients:

1 egg, beaten

½ cup finely grated mozzarella cheese

1 tbsp cream cheese, softened

1 tbsp sugar-free maple syrup

2 strawberries, sliced

2 raspberries, slices

¼ tsp blackberry extract

¼ tsp vanilla extract

½ cup plain yogurt for serving

Directions:

Preheat the waffle iron.

In a medium bowl, mix all the Ingredients except the yogurt.

Open the iron, lightly grease with Cooking spray and pour in a quarter of the mixture.

Close the iron and cook until golden brown and crispy, 7 minutes.

Remove the chaffle onto a plate and set aside.

Make three more chaffles with the remaining mixture.

To Servings: top with the yogurt and enjoy.

Nutrition:

Calories 78

Fats 5.29g carbs 3.02g net carbs 2.72g protein 4.32g

Ham and cheddar chaffles

Preparation   time: 15   minutes

Cooking   time: 28   minutes

Servings: 4

Ingredients:

1 cup finely shredded parsnips, steamed

8 oz ham, diced

2 eggs, beaten

1 ½ cups finely grated cheddar cheese

½ tsp garlic powder

2 tbsp chopped fresh parsley leaves

¼ tsp smoked paprika

½ tsp dried thyme

Salt and freshly ground black pepper to taste

Directions:

Preheat the waffle iron.

In a medium bowl, mix all the Ingredients. Open the iron, lightly grease with Cooking spray and pour in a quarter of the mixture. Close the iron and cook until crispy, 7 minutes. Remove the chaffle onto a plate and set aside. Make three more chaffles using the remaining mixture. Servings afterward.

Nutrition: Calories 506 Fats 24.05g carbs 30.02g net carbs 28.22g protein 42.74g

Savory gruyere and

chives chaffles

Preparation   time: 15   minutes

Cooking   time: 14   minutes

Servings: 2

Ingredients: 2 eggs, beaten

1 cup finely grated gruyere ch eese

2 tbsp finely grated cheddar cheese

1/8 tsp freshly ground black pepper

3 tbsp minced fresh chives + more for garnishing

2 sunshine fried eggs for topping

Directions:

Preheat the waffle iron.

In a medium bowl, mix the eggs, cheeses, black pepper, and chives.

Open the iron and pour in half of the mixture. Close the iron and cook until brown and crispy, 7 minutes. Remove the chaffle onto a plate and set aside.

Make another chaffle using the remaining mixture.

Top each chaffle with one fried egg each, garnish with the chives and Servings.

Nutrition: Calories 712 Fats 41.32g carbs 3.88g net carbs 3.78g protein 23.75g

Chicken quesadilla chaffle

Preparation time: 10 minutes

Cooking time: 14 minutes

Servings: 2

Ingredients:

1 egg, beaten

¼ tsp taco seasoning

1/3 cup finely grated cheddar cheese

1/3 cup cooked chopped chicken

Directions:

Preheat the waffle iron.

In a medium bowl, mix the eggs, taco seasoning, and cheddar cheese. Add the chicken and combine well.

Open the iron, lightly grease with Cooking spray and pour in half of the mixture.

Close the iron and cook until brown and crispy, 7 minutes.

Remove the chaffle onto a plate and set aside.

Make another chaffle using the remaining mixture.

Servings afterward.

Nutrition:

Calories 314

Fats 20.64g carbs 5.71g net carbs 5.71g protein 16.74g

Chicken jalapeno popper chaffle

Preparation time: 5 minutes

Cooking time: 5 minutes

Servings: 2

Ingredients 1/2 cup canned chicken breast

1/4 cup cheddar cheese

1/8 cup parmesan cheese - 1 egg

1 diced jalapeno (raw or pickled)

1/8 teaspoon onion powder

1/8 teaspoon of garlic powder

1 teaspoon of cream cheese

Directions: Preheat mini waffle maker.In an average bowl, add all Ingredients and stir together till it's completely incorporated.Half this mixture and pour a part of the mixture into a mini waffle maker and cook for a minimum of five minutes.

Note. Optional toppings: sour cream, ranch dressing, hot sauce, coriander, leek, feta cheese, jalapeno!

Nutritional value : Calories 224

Total fat 21.8g 34% Cholesterol 134.6mg 45%

Sodium 871mg 36%

Total carbohydrate 9.2g 3%

Dietary fiber 2.3g 9% Sugars 4.7g

Protein 18.5g 37% Vitamin a 163.1µg 11%

Vitamin c 0mg 0%

Crispy chaffle

Preparation time: 5 minutes s

Cooking time: 5 minutes

Servings: 2

Ingredients 2 eggs

1/2 cup parmesan cheese

Everything except 1 teaspoon bagel

1/2 cup mozzarella cheese

2 teaspoon almond flour

Directions:

Heat the mini waffle maker for about 30 seconds. Sprinkle the griddle with a range of cheese (i used parmesan and mozzarella cheese), melt and bake for 30 seconds, then add the mixture.

In a small bowl, add 2 eggs, 1 cup of cheese, 2 teaspoons of almond flour and bagel seasoning (if you are not a fan, you can skip the seasoning) and whisk.

Pour the mixture into a waffle maker so that it does not spill from the bottom.

Cook for 4 minutes (the longer the Cooking time, the quicker the crisper).

This mixture has two chaffles.

Nutritional value

Yield: 2 Servings, 1 serving: 1 crispy chaffle serving size: calories: 287, total carbohydrates: 6g, fiber: 0g, net carbohydrates: 6g, total fat: 20g, protein: 21g

Easy chicken parmesan chaffle

Preparation time: 5 minutes

Cooking time: 5 minutes

Servings: 2

Ingredients

Ingredients for chaffle:

1/2 cup of canned chicken breast or remaining shredded chicken

1/4 cup cheddar cheese

1/8 cup parmesan che ese

1 egg

1 teaspoon italian seasoning

1/8 teaspoon of garlic powder

1 teaspoon of cream cheese, room temperature

Topping Ingredients:

2 pieces of provolon cheese

1 tablespoon unsweetened pizza sauce

Directions:

Preheat the manufacturer of mini waffles.

In an average bowl, put together all the Ingredients and stir thoroughly until fully integrated.

Before putting together the mixture add one spoon of cheese (shredded) for few seconds to the waffle iron.

This will produce the best crust and making it easier to remove this heavy chaff from the waffle producer when it's done.

Add half of the mixture to the mini waffle maker and cook for at least 4 to 5 minutes.

Repeat the above moves to cook the second parmesan chicken chaffle.

While you slice the provolone, cheese add a sugar-free pizza sauce.

Tips

After Cooking a simple chicken parmesan chaffle, add it to a toaster oven, air fryer, or ninja foodi to make it crispy. Melt the cheese above to make this recipe special. It is worth the effort. You can also pop in the oven for a few minutes until the cheese melts and foa ms a little! Totally worth it!

Nutritional value

Calories 304

Total fat 21.8g 34%

Cholesterol 134.6mg 45%

Sodium 871mg 36%

Total carbohydrate 9.2g 3%

Dietary fiber 2.3g 9%

Sugars 4.7g

Protein 18.5g 37%

Vitamin a 163.1µg 11%

Vitamin c 0mg 0%